AF504884

Table of Contents

Making The Most Out Of Your Gym Time

A common goal most people usually write down for their new year's resolution is to lose weight. There will be a side note next to the goal saying how you'll be waking up every day at 5 am to go to your morning workout or how you will only eat vegetables and fruits and all that. While losing weight might be one of your goals, just writing it down and not doing anything about it for sure won't help your case. Two main things are effective when it comes to weight loss; nutrition and exercise. While we aren't going to talk so much about nutrition in this read, we are going to bring out the lowdown on exercise. Let's just see how many exercises per workout are needed for weight loss.

Going blindly to the gym and then jumping right into workouts might not give you the results you want. We give you the props for making an effort and making your way to the gym, but that is not all you need to do to lose weight. As the adage goes, failing to plan is planning to fail. Before you make your way to the gym, you need to have a plan; a plan that includes your goal and how to get to your goal. Your goal shouldn't be something general like, "I want to lose weight," have a specific number of pounds you want to lose. Something like I want to lose 20 pounds is more like it. Now since you know your goal, the next thing to do is to work towards it.

Nutrition without exercise is just giving nutrition a heavy burden to carry and vice versa. To lose weight, you need to do these things; check what you eat as you burn more calories at the gym.

Assuming you have the nutrition part in check, here are things you need to know to help yourself burn calories at the gym.

What Are The Factors That Influence Weight Loss?

There are certain factors apart from exercising and nutrition that affect weight loss that shouldn't be ignored. You might be hitting the gym as hard as you can, but your weight loss journey might be impaired without checking these factors. Here are some of these factors:

• **Sleep**

Sleep and weight loss go hand in hand. Sufficient sleep is required to promote weight loss. On average. a person should sleep for eight hours a day. Not getting enough sleep might have you starting bad habits like late night snacking, which will deter your weight loss journey. Studies also show that the less you sleep, the more likely you are to store fat and bring in more calories.

Apart from that, the lack of enough sleep also affects your hormones, and this can lead to weight gain. The hormones that are responsible for regulating your appetite are usually affected by the amount of sleep you get. These hormones are ghrelin and leptin. Ghrelin helps promote appetite and fat storage, while leptin helps to suppress your appetite. When you don't get enough sleep, this results in high levels of ghrelin and low levels of leptin, resulting in more food consumed.

- **Stress**

Stress is yet another thing that can affect your weight loss journey. The hormone associated with stress is cortisol. When your stress levels are high, your cortisol levels also increase. High levels of cortisol are usually responsible for reducing insulin sensitivity and can also promote the storage of fat around the stomach area. Stress also promotes habits like stress-eating, which results in you bringing in more calories than you normally do hence leading to weight gain.

- **Age**

The older you get, the more weight you are likely to gain. The main reason for this is the slowing of your metabolism. As you get older, most of your muscle mass starts being replaced by fat mass. It is known that muscles have a higher rate of metabolism at rest as compared to fat mass, so since your fat mass increases more than your muscle mass, your metabolism also reduces.

• Not Drinking Enough Water

Is there anyone who doesn't know the importance of drinking enough water? Well, here is another reason as to why you should drink enough water. Being hydrated helps prevent weight gain. When you are thirsty, your cells will signal to your brain that you need more fluid. The problem is that at times this signal isn't very clear to many people and they instead end up eating rather than drinking, which tends to promote weight gain

Apart from this, water helps in weight loss by promoting satiety. If you drink water before a meal, you are likely to feel full faster compared with not drinking water before eating. This reduces the calories you consume and thus promotes weight loss.

- **Genes**

Your genetic makeup also comes to play with issues related to weight gain and weight loss. Genes are known to affect the amount of fat your body stores and where it stores it. There are also some gene mutations that may cause an increase in appetite and weight gain.

How Many Exercises Per Workout Session For Weight Loss?

Just like most things when it comes to weight loss, there is no blanket answer to this question. There are factors that come into play, like how many pounds do you want to lose? Which kind of exercises are you doing? How long are you doing the exercises and so on.

When it comes to how many pounds you want to lose, the person who wants to lose more pounds will have to work out more than a person who wants to lose, let's say 2 pounds in 2 months.

When it comes to the kind of exercises you are doing, it goes without saying that different exercises burn calories differently. The number of calories you would burn doing mountain climbers is not the same number of calories you would burn by going for a walk.

When it comes to the intensity of the workout, the more intensity you put into your workout session, the more calories you are likely to burn. High-intensity workouts burn more calories than low or moderate intensity workouts.

How Much Should You Workout Everyday To Lose Weight?

When it comes to this question, we shall look at the two main exercises and how long you should do each in a week. The two main exercises that help with weight loss are cardiovascular exercises (aerobic activity) and strength training.

An average human being is advised to get a minimum of 150 minutes of moderate aerobic activity in a week or 75 minutes of vigorous aerobic activity or a mixture of the two. Since that is the amount that is advised for every week, you can divide those minutes by the number of times you workout every week. If you do vigorous aerobic activities 3 times a week, you need to do 25 minutes of vigorous aerobic exercises every workout session. If you do moderate aerobic activities 3 times a week, you need to do 50 minutes of moderate aerobic exercises every workout session. To have a clear difference between vigorous and moderate aerobic exercises, vigorous exercises include sprinting and jumping rope exercises. In contrast, moderate exercises include exercises like taking a walk and swimming.

When it comes to strength training, an average human is advised to do strength training for all the major muscle groups for a minimum of two times a week. You are also advised to at least do a single set for each exercise. You should use a resistance that is heavy enough to tire your muscles after 12 to 15 repetitions. When it comes to resistance training, you can use your own bodyweight or use resistance equipment like resistance bands.

It goes without saying, but the more you exercise, the faster you are to getting to your weight goals. If you feel like 150 minutes of moderate cardio are not enough, ramp up your exercise and do 200 minutes or even 300 minutes. Being active also helps to lose weight, so try as much as you can to be up and going instead of sitting curled on the sofa watching a tv series for more than 6 hours.

How Many Calories Should You Burn In A Workout To Lose Weight?

In order to lose weight, you have to burn more calories than you consume. The recommended weight loss is 1 – 2 pounds in a week. That translates to 3500 to 7000 calories in a week. So, if you are trying to lose 1 pound in a week, you have to divide it between eating fewer calories and working out. A good way to do this is to lose 1500 calories by cutting your calorie intake and 2000 calories from working out in a week.

If you only workout 5 days a week because you don't want to work out every day of the week (as rest is also important in a workout program), you need to burn 400 to 500 calories in each workout. This translates to 2000 calories, and as a result you are going to be able to hit your weekly target. You need to keep in mind that the number of calories you burn is influenced by things like weight, gender and other factors. A man who is 180 pounds is likely to burn more calories than a woman who weighs 120 pounds while both doing the same workout.

How To Track The Calories You Burn Per Workout?

The good thing about technology is that it has made things like tracking calories easier. The Apple Watch and many other smartwatches can help you track the number of calories you burn while working out.

Apart from using the smartwatches, you can use various online calculators that help track the calories you burn in a workout:

The online calculators use this formula to calculate how many calories you burn per workout:

Calories Burned = Duration of the exercise in minutes * (MET * 3.5 * Weight in Kgs)/200

MET, also referred to as the metabolic equivalent for a task, estimates how much energy your body uses during a certain activity, and all online calculators have this built-in.

How Many Exercises Per Workout Session For Weight Loss

Since there is no exact answer that would be sufficient for everyone, below is a table highlighting the calories a 125-pound person, a 155-pound person and a 185-pound person are likely to burn doing different workouts for 30 minutes (2).

CALORIES BURNED IN HALF AN HOUR

ACTIVITY	125 POUND PERSON	155 POUND PERSON	185 POUND PERSON
General Weight Lifting	90	112	133
Water Aerobics	120	149	178
Stretching, Hatha Yoga	120	149	178
Moderate Calisthenics	135	167	200
General Riders	150	186	222
Low Impact Aerobics	165	205	244
General Stair Step Machine	180	223	266
Teaching Aerobics	180	223	266
Vigorous Weight Lifting	180	223	266
Low Impact Aerobics, Step	210	260	311
High Impact Aerobics	210	260	311

To determine how many exercises per workout for weight loss, you need to first set your daily goal, which is the amount of calories you need to burn per day. With that done, depending on the weight category you belong to from the table, you can be able to see how many calories you burn from doing the different exercises and sporting activities. For the people in the intermediate weights which are not mentioned, you can use the weight close to your weight to approximate the number of calories you are likely to burn from the workout as the numbers don't differ by large numbers. For example, if you are 160 pounds, you can use the 155 pound table.

Using Planks To Shed Off Some Extra Pounds

Weight loss is important as it helps prevent certain health conditions like diabetes and various heart conditions. This is one of the reasons why people who are overweight are advised to lose weight. There are different ways to do so, and these methods are affected by factors like age, current weight, gender, genes, amount of sleep, stress levels of the person, and others. Two of the most recommended ways of losing weight are cutting on calories and working out. Different exercises can help with weight loss, and that is why we shall look at planking for weight loss in this read.

What Is A Plank?

A plank is an exercise that works to help strengthen the core by working the transversus abdominis muscle. This muscle is responsible for supporting and stabilizing the torso during isometric contractions. A plank is also said to be a workout that helps strengthen the core in general and the abdomen area. Since the main purpose of a plank is to strengthen your core, it is therefore responsible for improving your posture, which helps reduce back-related injuries and lower back pains.

The plank is known for working the muscles around the core area, but those are not the only muscles it works on, as it targets most major muscles too, including various leg muscles and hand muscles. Planks are pretty famous as most workout plans have to involve either the traditional plank or its variation. Variations of the plank are usually for people who have mastered the art of doing the basic plank, and they feel like they need to make the plank a little bit challenging for themselves.

Planks are also famous for the fact that they provide substantial results for a short period. It belongs to the strength training group of workouts because they help build strength, and this means they do not burn a lot of calories, but that does not mean they don't help in weight loss as you will see how they aid in weight loss in later parts of this read.

How To Do A Plank?

It is important to know how to do a plank properly because this enables you to enjoy all the benefits associated with this exercise. Just like any other exercise, maintaining the right form while doing a plank is very important as it prevents various injuries that might be associated with doing it wrong. With that said, here is how you do a plank:

1. You start by kneeling on your yoga mat or whatever you are using to prevent your elbows from getting injured.

2. The next step is to place your elbows on the mat.

3. Then with your legs hip-width apart, extend your right leg back and then your left leg.

4. While doing all this, make sure to keep your neck, back, and hips in the same line and your core engaged.

5. Hold this pose for at least 10 seconds.

6. You should do 3 sets of 10 to 30 seconds hold.

Common Mistakes Done When Doing A Plank

There are mistakes that most beginners make when doing planks. This is bad as it increases their risks of getting injuries. Here are some of these mistakes:

Collapsing Your Lower Back

You find most people risk getting back pains while doing planks by dipping their butts. This removes the torso from the flat position it should be in, putting a strain on your spinal cord and increasing the risk of back pains. To prevent this from happening and to help you to maintain the right body positions while doing a plank, you can ask a colleague or a person at the gym to place a stick on your back. At all times, make sure the top of the stick is touching your head and the bottom rests between your buttocks. It should also make contact right between your shoulder blades for proper alignment.

Tilting Your Head Up

When you are doing a plank, your neck, back, and hips should be in a straight line. Your neck should not be tilted up, as this could strain your neck, which is something you don't want.

Planking For Weight Loss: Moving Your Butt Upwards

Your butt shouldn't be in a position higher than the back or a position similar to the downward dog when doing planks . This prevents the body from engaging the core as it should during the plank. The aim is to keep your back and your butt flat enough so that your abs are engaged. While doing this, make sure you don't dip your butt too much either.

Letting Your Head Drop

This is more common to happen. This usually happens when the person starts to check the rest of the other body parts, like the stomach, while doing the plank. While they may be checking to see if the other body parts are in the right position, they may forget to return their head to the needed position, resulting in a poor form of doing the exercise.

Sagging Your Hips

Your hips usually start sinking when your abs have gotten tired, and this should be a clear sign that it is time to end your plank. If you notice your hips are sinking right from the start of the exercise, try to separate your feet a bit wider and focus on engaging your abs.

Not Breathing

As humans, we hold our breaths while we are in a strenuous position, which is not advisable, especially while doing a plank. This restricts the amount of oxygen getting into your body, and this can cause nausea or dizziness.

Focusing Too Much On Your Stopwatch

This can be your stopwatch or whatever instrument you are using to measure the time you spend on the plank. You need to know when to stop as doing a plank for long in a bad form does not really help, and that is just tiring yourself for no reason.

Arching Your Back

When you are doing a plank and arching your back at the same time, you are not engaging your abdominal muscles as you should. Instead, you are putting more weight on your hands. To prevent this from happening, always make sure your shoulders are wide and down.

How Long Should You Hold A Plank For Weight Loss?

It goes without saying that the longer you hold the plank, the more calories you burn. The question is, can you really hold a plank for that long while maintaining the right form? The plank is not the easiest of exercises, and just like any other exercise, you get better at it the more you do it.

According to experts, the length of time you can hold a plank can vary from 10 seconds to 60 seconds. Well, it's hard for a beginner who started planking today to hold a plank for 60 seconds, and that's why if you are new to the exercise, you are advised to start with shorter reps as you work yourself up the ladder. Short plank holds are also an effective workout, and you should not think that the only way you can get the most out of a plank is by doing it for a long time.

Planking For Weight Loss

If you are a beginner, start by holding a plank for 10 seconds, and rest for about 5 to 10 seconds, then do another plank for another 10 seconds. Repeat this for 3 to 6 sets. By doing this, you can receive the same strength benefits you would have gotten for holding the plank for 30 seconds or 60 seconds continuously as you are still working your muscles for the same amount of total time. If you are a pro and 60 minutes just doesn't do it for you anymore, you can increase the difficulty of doing the plank by contracting your abs more, squeezing your glutes more, and squeezing your quads more. You can also try different variations of the plank that are a bit harder and more intense.

When holding a plank, it is always important to listen to your body, even if you plan to hold it for a long time. Your body will tell you when to stop. If you try to hold a plank longer than you actually can, you put yourself at risk of getting injured. The more tired you get, the more your back starts to arch, which increases your chances of getting injured while doing the exercise or may cause lower back pains.

Who Should Not Do A Plank?

Although a plank is recommended for all people, certain groups of people shouldn't attempt it. These people are:

People With Shoulder Injuries

The plank engages your shoulders too much. If you have a shoulder injury, doing a plank would only make the situation worse.

People Who Feel Pain On Their Shoulders After The Exercise

Planks should make you feel a lot of things, but the pain in the shoulders is not a good sign. If you feel pain on the shoulders after doing a plank, you should consult an expert before you do the exercise again.

Pregnant Women

Expectant mothers are usually advised to exercise, but planks are not one of those that they should be doing. First and foremost, the plank position does not give the mother enough room to actually perform the exercise. Secondly, doing the workout might cause the mother to fall, which might cause injuries and even worse things; hence, if you are an expectant mother, you should steer clear planks.

People Who Have Been Told By An Expert Not To Do Them

If an expert tells you not to do a plank, then you should listen to them as they have a reason as to why they are telling you that.

People Who Don't Know The Right Form Of Doing A Plank

If you don't know how to do a plank correctly, you shouldn't be doing the plank, to begin with, as this increases the chances of you getting injured.

Planking And Weight Loss

As mentioned earlier, planking is a strength training exercise, and thus it does not burn as many calories as exercises belonging to cardiovascular exercises such as jump rope do. This does, however, not mean that planks cannot help you lose weight. Although they don't burn as many calories as cardiovascular exercises, they burn some calories, which does help with weight loss. If you are 150 pounds and do a plank for one minute, you will likely burn approximately 3 calories.

Another way planks help with weight loss is by building strength. Although planks are not good at burning calories, they are actually good when it comes to building muscles, which goes a long way in helping burn calories. Muscles have a high resting metabolism compared to fat mass. This means they burn more calories at rest compared to fat. This helps a person burn calories and thus leads to weight loss. Therefore, we can say planks help with weight loss by building muscles.

Benefits Of Planking

Apart from helping with weight loss, planks have other benefits they offer. Here are some of these benefits:

• Planks Help Build Strength – Planking For Weight Loss

Planks are part of strength training exercises and thus help build strength and muscles. Being strong is helpful in many ways. Being strong makes everyday activities like carrying groceries from the car to the house easy.

• Planks Are A Full-Body Workout

Despite the belief that planks mostly work out the core muscles, the planks actually engage muscles all over the body, from the neck all the way to the legs. When done properly, planks work your glutes, quads, triceps, lats, biceps, etc.

• Planks Work And Improve Your Core's Performance

Planks are an effective exercise when it comes to working the core because they engage all of its muscles. These are muscles like the transverse abdominis, rectus abdominis, oblique muscles, and glutes. Having a strong core helps in so many ways. A strong core helps with movements as all the various limbs' movements originate from the core. A strong core also helps stabilize, balance, and power the body during the various activities you do during the day. This helps prevent fall injuries. A strong core also makes everyday activities like sitting on the desk all day, putting on your shoes, or standing become easier.

• Planks Help Reduce The Risk Of Back And Spinal Column Injuries

Planks help you build muscle all over the body while also making sure you don't put a lot of pressure on your spine and back. Planking regularly helps build back muscles, and these muscles form a strong support for your entire back. This also helps prevent back pains.

• Planks Help Improve Your Posture – Planking For Weight Loss

Nobody wants to have a bad posture. Planks, by making the core strong, help improve your posture. A good posture helps keep both your joints and bones in the correct alignment, and this helps both of them to be better maintained and healthy. It also helps prevent backaches and pains and makes a person look better and feel more confident.

• Planks Help Improve Your Flexibility

The form you hold while doing planks helps with stretching all your posterior muscle groups and this helps improve your flexibility. When you are flexible, you perform better when it comes to physical activities, you are less prone to injuries, and you have a good posture.

The Bottom Line

Planking for weight loss requires you to build muscles so you can increase your resting metabolism, and hence promote weight loss. Planks are not cardiovascular exercises, which is why they do not burn so many calories. While doing a plank, it is always important to remember to hold the correct form. Doing this exercise in the wrong form can cause injuries very easily. Do not try to hold a plank for longer if you can't, as you are likely to compromise on your form. Short plank holds have the same benefits as long plank holds. Do what you can and go on adding the number of seconds you can hold a plank when you get used to the exercise. If you have any existing shoulder injuries or an expert has instructed you not to do planks, you should not attempt to do them.